GETTING
STARTED
WITH
Aromatherapy

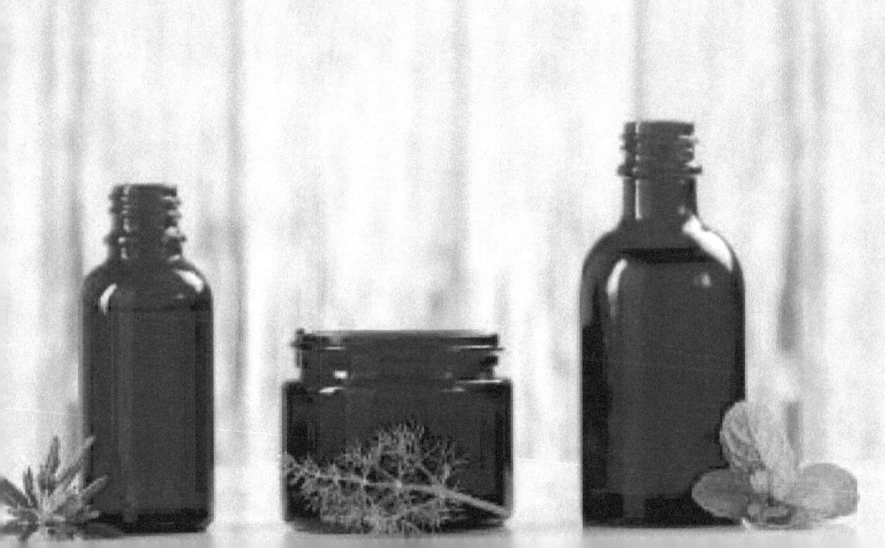

Getting Started With Aromatherapy

Table of Contents

Introduction

Aromatherapy uses aromas to enhance physiological and psychological well-being. It also includes the use of complementary ingredients that are found in nature. A few include:

- The use of sugar as an exfoliate

- Clays and muds to purify the skin

- Sea salts

- Herbs

- Cold-pressed vegetable oils

Aromatherapy has been in existence for thousands of years, but the distillation process required to extract essential oils wasn't developed until the 11th century. Aromatherapy enjoys popularity in the United States, India, England, and France.

There can be much more involved in aromatherapy than smelling a few essential oils. The use of herbal distillates, carrier oils, vaporizer oils and phytoncides can make aromatherapy quite complex!

Fortunately, it isn't necessary to make aromatherapy complex. The beginner can enjoy the benefits of aromatherapy with simple methods.

The aromas used in aromatherapy are acquired from two sources:

1. **Plant extracts.** Extracts are obtained by either cold pressing the plants or soaking the plants in a volatile liquid.

   - Extracts may be used in aromatherapy, but have other uses, too. For example, vanilla extract is used in cooking and other extracts are used as insect repellent.

2. **Plant essential oils.** Using a distillation process, the water portion is removed. The small amount of oil that remains is the essential oil.

   - A large quantity of plant material is necessary to produce a small amount of essential oil. The quantity of plant material needed, and the energy required to perform the distillation explain the typically higher price of essential oils versus extracts.

- Essential oils are primarily used for therapeutic purposes.

Keep in mind that essential oils differ from the fragrance oils found in perfumes. Fragrance oils can contain artificial ingredients and lack the therapeutic action of essential oils. **The use of synthetic ingredients is not encouraged in aromatherapy.**

If you're looking for a natural way to treat common physical and psychological issues, aromatherapy might be beneficial to you.

"I mix all different oils – my bathroom at home is littered with oils; I'm really into natural beauty and natural healing.

Peppermint is really good if you put it on your stomach for a tummy ache; lavender is kind of all-purpose - I think everyone should carry it."

- Liz Goldwyn

Aromatherapy Benefits

Several studies have shown that aromatherapy provides benefits. **The markers for the scent molecules have been found in the blood of patients after aromatherapy treatment, suggesting that the potential for advantageous effects exist.** That's exciting news!

Studies have shown that many animals can be calmed or agitated by essential oils. Behavior and immune responses are strengthened. There is no doubt that essential oils have antimicrobial properties when administered to the skin.

As you would expect, many in the medical community are skeptical and poorly informed. However, that can be expected to change over time.

Aromatherapy provides several unique benefits:

1. **Strengthens the immune system.** Prevention is preferable to a cure when it comes to sickness! Aromatherapy is believed to have antibacterial and antifungal effects.

Many studies have been conducted on this aspect of aromatherapy use.

2. **Reduces anxiety and depression.** The reduction of stress and anxiety is the most popular use of aromatherapy. Most beginners in aromatherapy focus on stress reduction. Stress is a common challenge, and the application of aromatherapy for this purpose can be simple, yet still effective.

   • **Depression relief is the second most common usage of aromatherapy.** The drugs used to treat depression can also provide a lot of side effects. Aromatherapy can be a helpful addition of psychological counseling and avoids the negative aspects of pharmaceutical therapy.

3. **Boosts energy levels.** Aromatherapy is often used as an energy booster. Life is hectic and a higher level of energy can be useful!

4. **Aid in sleep quality.** Essential oils are used to realign circadian rhythms and to help

balance sleep schedules.

5. **Facilitates the healing process.** Proponents of aromatherapy claim it can speed healing throughout the body. Aromatherapy can increase the blood flow and the amount of oxygen that reaches a wound. It is also used after surgery.

6. **Eliminates pain.** Aromatherapy can help to alleviate pain, particularly the pain caused by headaches. While the pain is addressed directly, it can also be lessened by the reduction of stress and anxiety that aromatherapy provides.

7. **Enhances cognitive performance.** Memory has been shown to be enhanced with the use of aromatherapy. However, the effect seems to be limited in duration.

8. **Enhances digestion.** Aromatherapy is also used for issues with bloating, indigestion, and constipation.

It's easy to see that aromatherapy has the ability to ease many physical and psychological conditions.

Aromatherapy makes good use of the idea of synergy. **The skillful combining of several essential oils is believed to provide greater results than single oils.** The presence of one oil can enhance the strength of another.

"Aromatherapy is a caring, hands-on therapy which seeks to induce relaxation, to increase energy, to reduce the effects of stress and to restore lost balance to mind, body and soul."

- Robert Tisserand

What is Needed to Begin Using Aromatherapy?

Maybe you've developed an interest in aromatherapy, but are wondering how to get started. For the beginner, aromatherapy can be overwhelming. Where do you even begin?

It can also be expensive. It doesn't have to be expensive, but the potential to spend a lot of money is there. It's important to figure out what you require and what can wait for another day. Some purchases don't have to be made immediately.

To get started, you have two primary options:

1. Purchase a kit.
2. Build your own kit.

It's hard to make a mistake by purchasing a kit. However, you're likely to end up with some things you'll never use. You're also likely to want an essential oil that isn't included.

It's also more fun to build your own kit! You'll learn a lot along the way, too.

Consider these tips to build your own aromatherapy kit:

1. **Determine the essential oils you'll need.** You can do some research and come to your own conclusions. These oils are very popular, and some of the least expensive:

   - Roman Chamomile – *Chamaemelum nobile*
   - Eucalyptus – *Eucalyptus globulus*
   - Frankincense – Boswellia carterii
   - Lavender – *Lavandula angustifolia*
   - Lemon – *Citrus limon*
   - Orange – *Citrus sinensis*
   - Peppermint – *Mentha piperita*
   - Rosemary – *Rosmarinus officinalis*
   - Sandalwood - *Santalum album*
   - Tea Tree – *Melaleuca alternifolia*

2. **Choose your carrier oils.** Remember that carriers are used to dilute the essential oils. They also allow the essential oils to be applied

to your skin. Recommendations for beginners include:

- Fragrance free lotion
- Jojoba oil
- Almond oil
- Liquid Castile soap.
    - This soap is made from olive oil and sodium hydroxide. It is free from animal fats, unlike many other types of soaps. It's considered to be eco-friendly and biodegradable.

3. **Storage supplies.** You'll want to store your lotions and potions in a convenient manner. There are several types of containers you're likely to need.

- Amber glass bottles. These can be small. 5ml to 15 ml is sufficient. Ensure that the bottles are amber, rather than clear. **Light can degrade some essential oils.**

- Glass jars to store your lotions. A 2 oz. glass jar with a wide mouth is perfect. Two ounces equals a quarter of a cup.

- Plastic spray bottles. Avoid purchasing anything too large. Bottles between 2 oz. and 4 oz. are fine.

- Blank nasal inhalers. If you remember the old style of Vick's inhalers, these are similar. They are commonly sold in 10- or 12-packs.

4. **Miscellaneous.** A few glass beakers or flasks and a glass rod or two are convenient for mixing oils. You'll also need:

- A record keeping system. A notebook is the easiest way to record your recipes, thoughts, and results.

- A labeling system. You can purchase a label maker or resort to a ballpoint pen and masking tape. It's up to you.

- Storage. A dedicated work space is ideal, but just a dream for many. A plastic storage tub can be an effective second choice.

Building your own aromatherapy kit might seem a bit intimidating, but there are many online resources. Books on the topic are as close as your nearest library or bookstore.

You might consider purchasing a kit and filling in the gaps with additional supplies. **A limited budget doesn't have to be an obstacle.** A couple of essential oils are all that you need to get started.

"The art of healing comes from nature, not from the physician. Therefore, the physician must start from nature, with an open mind."

- Paracelsus

Safety

Essential oils are chemicals. **As with any other chemical, the potential for danger exists.** It's important to understand what you're doing before inhaling any substance or putting it directly onto your skin.

The hazards are easily avoided, but you must understand the hazards before you can expect to avoid them.

Always be safe while performing aromatherapy:

1. **Some essential oils can exacerbate certain conditions.** Certain oils should be avoided by those with existing medical conditions, such as asthma, epilepsy, and pregnancy. It's important to be aware of this issue. To ensure you're being safe, perform the necessary research on the oils you might like to try.

2. **Avoid applying essential oils directly to the skin without diluting them first.** Two common examples of exceptions include

17

lavender and tea tree, but there are still risks. It's much easier to develop sensitivities to specific oils when they are applied in high concentrations.

3. **Some oils react with ultraviolet light, specifically UVA.** These exposed oils can then cause blistering and redness to the skin. **The primary culprits are cold-pressed citrus oils.** The distilled citrus oils are generally considered to be safe when exposed to UVA. **Other phototoxic essential oils include:**

    *   Angelica Root Essential Oil
    *   Bergamot (Cold Pressed)
    *   Bitter Orange (Cold Pressed)
    *   Cumin
    *   Fig Leaf Absolute
    *   Grapefruit (Cold Pressed)
    *   Lemon (Cold Pressed)
    *   Lime (Cold Pressed)
    *   Mandarin Leaf

4. **Essential oils can lead to allergic reactions or other types of sensitivities.** It's a good idea to test any oils you've never used before on a small patch of skin.

- **To test for sensitivity, dilute the essential oil in question to a 2% concentration.** The quick and dirty way to do this is to add 12 drops of essential oil to 30 ml of carrier oil or lotion. One tablespoon equals 15 ml.

- Put one drop of the diluted oil on your skin. The arm is a good location.

- Put a band aid or similar bandage over the oil and wait. If you feel any discomfort within 24 hours, immediately wash the area with soap and water.

- If 24 hours pass without any negative reaction, you can consider the oil safe to use on your skin.

5. **Some essential oils are considered unsafe for use by non-experts.** A few of these

include: camphor, onion, wintergreen and bitter almond. There are more complete lists available online.

6. **Beware of mixing aromatherapy and children.** Young children are curious and love the smell of many aromatherapy mixtures. This often results in the child drinking the mixture. **Treat aromatherapy solutions as poisons when children are involved.** Avoid underestimating the ability of your child to surprise you.

7. **Do not consume essential oils.** Your child shouldn't be drinking them, and neither should you! Though many oils are derived from common foods, essential oils are highly concentrated and can cause severe damage when misused like this.

Essential oils have the power to heal and to harm. Understand the dangers that essential oils can pose in certain situations. Avoid causing yourself any undue harm.

Remember, you're trying to bring comfort to yourself, not create additional suffering in your life. Use aromatherapy wisely.

"I believe that for every illness or ailment known to man, that God has a plant out here that will heal it. We just need to keep discovering the properties for natural healing."

- Vannoy Gentles Fite

How to Use Essential Oils

There are a variety of ways to use essential oils. You might even be able to come up with a few on your own.

Just remember to be alert for signs of sensitivity whenever introducing a new oil to your regimen. And of course, avoid consuming the oils!

Use a method of administration that works for your situation:

1. **Inhale the scent directly.** This is the easiest way to get started. Place a couple of drops of the essential oil on a tissue or paper towel. Hold the tissue close to your face and inhale through your nose.

2. **Bath.** Just 5 drops in one ounce of carrier oil, such as almond oil, can be added to your bath water. Ensure that you're choosing an appropriate essential oil.

3. **Inhale via steam.** Boil two cups of water and then transfer the water to a bowl. Add approximately five drops of essential oil to the water. Keep the bowl close to you and enjoy the scent. Stop if you experience any discomfort.

4. **The room method.** Follow the previous method, but use 10 drops of essential oil. Place the bowl near the center of the room. The goal is to fill the room with the aroma of the essential oil.

5. **Massage.** Add 10-20 drops of essential oil to 1/8 cup of carrier oil. Almond or jojoba oil are acceptable carrier oils. Ideally, have a partner massage the oil into your skin. Stay away from the eyes and mucous membranes.

6. **Other.** Essential oils can be used to make many household products, such as soap, shampoo, lotions, and shower gel.

Try all the different methods and see which works the best for you.

There's no method that is universally superior to another. Keep an open mind and experiment. You'll likely find one method that you prefer over the others.

"Healing is a matter of time, but it is sometimes also a matter of opportunity."

\- Hippocrates

Aromatherapy Devices

You might be wondering if there is a better way of enjoying your essential oils than applying your mixtures to a tissue or a hot bowl of water. You're in luck! Most of them are relatively inexpensive, too.

There are several devices that can be used to enjoy your essential oils more conveniently:

1. **Diffusers.** You don't need a carrier oil with a diffuser. Just add water to the diffuser and then add your essential oils. The ultrasonic action releases the mixture into the air. Diffusers come in a variety of sizes. Most are sufficient for a large room for up to 8 hours.

   - Some diffusers have an elegant appearance and include various color-changing modes. Ensure that you examine your options and find a diffuser that matches your tastes and décor.

2. **Nebulizer.** This is a special type of diffuser. It works very quickly and uses a highly pressurized air stream to break the essential

oils into tiny particles and inject them into the air. Nebulizers are more expensive, but more effective than conventional diffusers.

3. **Heaters.** You've undoubtedly noticed how the smell of hot chocolate-chip cookies can fill your household, yet the smell seems to vanish when the cookies cool. There are heaters designed specifically to heat your aromatherapy oils. These work slowly but effectively.

- There are even aromatherapy heater-alarm clocks! It can be used to provide calming scents at bedtime or when it's time to wake up.

"Nothing is more memorable than a smell. One scent can be unexpected, momentary and fleeting, yet conjure up a childhood summer beside a lake in the mountains."

- Diane Ackerman

Recipes

There are enough aromatherapy recipes to keep you busy for a lifetime. Again, keep an open mind and try a new recipe or two each week.

You'll soon notice that certain oils appeal to you while others clearly do not. Over time, you'll develop a catalog of recipes that work well for you.

Here are just a few to try…

Anxiety reduction bath oil:

- 9 drops of sandalwood
- 6 drops of orange
- 20 drops of lavender
- 2 fluid ounces of jojoba
- This mixture can be stored in a glass bottle.
- This recipe is enough for 8 baths. Avoid using it all at once!

Depression-reducing massage oil:

- 2 drops rose

- 6 drops sandalwood

- 2 drops orange

- 1 fluid ounce of almond oil

- Feel free to double or triple the recipe. Remember that a little goes a long way.

- The remainder can be stored in a glass container. Protect from light.

Sleep peacefully blend:

- 10 drops of roman chamomile

- 5 drops of bergamot

- 5 drops of clary sage

- Add 1 or 2 drops to a tissue and place inside your pillowcase.

Romance diffuser blend:

- 3 drops of orange oil

- 2 drops of Ylang Ylang oil

- Add these to your diffuser of choice,
  following the instructions for your diffuser.

There are an endless number of recipes online. **Do a little research and find a few blends that intrigue you.**

A word of warning: you'll often be missing one key ingredient! Find a local source of essential oils and you'll always be prepared.

"To be honest, I didn't really understand how involved putting a fragrance together could be - or would be. Once I made the choice to actually do it, I just went for it. I just dove in and have really learned a lot about putting a scent together. It's kind of exciting"

– Faith Hill

Conclusion

Aromatherapy has been around since at least the time of the Egyptians. The development of steam distillation took this science to another level overnight.

In modern times, scientific studies have shown the efficacy of aromatherapy in the treatment of many disorders and symptoms.

Before using aromatherapy, it's important to understand the safety implications. Anything that has the ability to heal can also potentially cause harm.

Treat aromatherapy like any other drug, because that's precisely what it is. Avoid experimenting until you have a solid understanding of aromatherapy in general.

You now have a basic understanding of aromatherapy and the benefits. You can acquire the necessary supplies to get started, but continue to learn more about aromatherapy. There are entire books written on single aromatherapy topics.

Keep learning and you'll discover that, with essential oils and aromatherapy, there's a whole new world out there with benefits that you never realized existed!

www.ingramcontent.com/pod-product-compliance
Lightning Source LLC
Chambersburg PA
CBHW051407280526
45784CB00007B/3141